Beating the Sugar B.E.A.S.T.

Lifestyle Management for People of Color Living with Diabetes

ISBN: 978-0-578-28140-7

Acknowledgments

This book would not have become a reality without the sacrifices made by my family, Arvel, Joshua and Camden. I am forever grateful to you all for making sure I made deadlines, allowed time for me to attend meetings, calls and encouraging me along the way.

To Michelle Greene Rhodes and my RNterprise Family; thanks for pushing me, encouraging me and cheering me on throughout this process. Appreciate the camaraderie, sisterhood and support system that continues to push me to the next level of my career.

Table of Contents

My Why

Beating the Sugar B.E.A.S.T. Lifestyle Management for People of Color Living with Diabetes has been at the forefront of my mind for some time. I've known for a while that it was part of my mission and purpose to share educational tips on management techniques. During the past 20+ years of practicing as a Registered Nurse, I have taken care of, provided education to and unfortunately witnessed the devastating effects of diabetes complications in people of color all too often. Diabetes is a chronic, lifelong condition that can be treated and managed effectively through different treatment modalities but, at the end of the day, each person plays a role in his or her own journey of controlling and managing the condition.

Unfortunately, the initial diagnosis of diabetes does not always mean change for some. For some people when the diagnosis is received, they do everything they can to lose weight and get their blood sugar numbers under better control. Meanwhile, others do not make any changes to their lifestyles and continue in their previous dietary habits and lack of/extremely limited physical activity. Because of this, they are now also dealing with a multitude of other medical diagnoses. Throughout the book, there are discussions about changes that can be made immediately while understanding that this is not an overnight event. Improvement will take time. As the saying goes, slow and steady wins the race. Diabetes management is more about consistency and staying the course as much as possible rather than finding a quick fix. Beating the Sugar B.E.A.S.T. is a daily endeavor, but one that can be completed

CHAPTER 1:

Introduction

In the United States, 96 million adults (more than 1 in 3) are living with prediabetes. This means that they have blood sugar levels that are higher than normal. The worst part is that if left untreated and if the current habits are maintained, these adults will develop Type 2 diabetes. Most people who have prediabetes are unaware that anything is even wrong. You won't necessarily feel any symptoms if you have high blood sugar, and so it's unlikely that you'd take any action to make significant lifestyle changes. Diabetes is a disorder in which the body is unable to either make enough insulin or to use it effectively. When this is the case, the result is consistently high blood glucose levels. Over time, high blood sugar can cause some very serious health problems including heart or kidney disease and vision loss.

We've all probably known someone who has been diagnosed with diabetes, but we tend to assume that it won't happen to us. There is a strong genetic component to diabetes, but it is also inextricably linked to our habits and lifestyle. Unfortunately, however, we've adopted a lifestyle based on the habits of those around us. If we grew up in a family where many of our family members were living with diabetes, we likely have the same habits ingrained in us as part of our upbringing. In other words, the stage is set, and most of us blindly accept our fate. We decide that we will maintain our current lifestyle for as long as we can and will deal with the consequences of that lifestyle when or if they come.

Or perhaps, we do know better. We might be very aware that we're making poor choices, but due to various socioeconomic factors, we find ourselves forced to make tough choices. This might mean we decide to keep the lights on instead of paying extra to acquire healthier, more expensive food. Perhaps we pay the rent instead of purchasing needed medication. Or maybe we have to cancel a gym membership because oil prices are rising, and we have to cut corners wherever we can. Sometimes life does come with hard choices, and our circumstances play their role in dictating how we respond. The good news is that we may not be able to change our current circumstances, but we always have choices. As long as we have free will, we have the ability to improve our circumstances and take charge of our own health. The little decisions that we make every day can be the difference between a life of health or one riddled with illness.

The first step is always going to be awareness. Once we are aware of how our daily choices affect our health, we then have the ability to make changes. That's where a lot of our family members may have gotten lost. Many of them never knew that what foods they chose to eat or how much they chose to exercise affected their future health to such a large extent. We can't rely on outside forces to guide us. Instead, we have to take things into our own hands and be our own advocates. Once we know there is a better way, we have to search for information and advice to support us on a healthier lifestyle.

It's very do-able, and this book is meant to make things even easier. Diabetes is not a death sentence. It can be successfully managed with healthy lifestyle choices. The truth, however, is that it can be more difficult for people of color because there are additional socioeconomic forces that come into play. For many individuals, "eating healthier" sounds like a pipe dream because they live in a food desert, where there really is no choice. What then?

What we cannot do is give up. There is always a way. The hurdles in front of us mean that we have to get a little more creative. Many of us, whether living in a food desert or not, have a cell phone. That connection to the Internet in your pocket can be your key to health. With it, you can order food online based on your budgetary allowances, track your daily activity, and even continue your education so you can move out of that food desert.

The guidance that you will find in this book will help you if you're someone who is already trying to manage diabetes or if you have not yet been diagnosed but are at risk. The changes that I advise are beneficial for everyone. Every member of your family stands to gain by making the changes I lay out here. By living in this way, those who are healthy today can secure a future where they continue to be healthy. The advice I give in this book is ideal for managing diabetes, but it also is the same recipe that could help a person avoid heart disease, high blood pressure, obesity, stroke and other chronic illnesses. In that respect, the B.E.A.S.T methodology is a simple framework for a brighter future.

Thoughts to Ponder:

- Do you know your fasting blood glucose number?

- Do you know your Hba1c percentage?

- What risk factors do you have for Prediabetes or Type 2 diabetes?

CHAPTER 2:

What is Diabetes?

There are three types of diabetes. Type 1 diabetes is thought to be caused by an autoimmune reaction that stops your body from making insulin. You can get type 1 diabetes at any age, but it usually develops in children, teens, or young adults. If you have Type 1 diabetes, you will have to receive insulin daily to help your body handle glucose and for you to survive.

Type 2 Diabetes typically occurs later in life but, more and more children, teens and young adults are being diagnosed. In Type 2 diabetes, your body has lost the ability to properly utilize insulin or has become resistant to it, which results in high blood sugar levels. These elevated levels have the potential to damage other systems within the body. About 90-95% of people with diabetes have this type.

The third type of diabetes is gestational diabetes. This develops in pregnant women who have had no previous history of diabetes. Gestational diabetes usually goes away after pregnancy but is associated with greater risk of Type 2 diabetes in the future.

When it comes to the numbers, diabetes seems to turn up more often in American Indians/Alaska Natives (14.7%), Hispanics (12.5%) and non-Hispanic blacks (11.7%). Another interesting fact to note is that prevalence seems to vary significantly by education level, which is an indicator that socioeconomic status plays a role. According to the National Diabetes Statistical Report 2020 Estimates of Diabetes and Its Burden in the United States, 13.3% of adults with less than a high school education developed diabetes as opposed to 9.7% of those with a high school education and 7.5% of those with more than a high school education.

The question then becomes how could a disease associated with blood sugar levels affect those with less education more often. The answer in my opinion has to do with opportunity and resources. When individuals are on a limited budget, they are forced to make different choices in terms of diet. Healthier foods tend to be more expensive and in many areas are completely inaccessible. When individuals are working many jobs to make ends meet while simultaneously raising a family, there often isn't time to cook healthy meals. Instead, they are forced to eat whatever is quick, easy and accessible. These meals may contain high amounts of sugar, salt, fried foods and processed ingredients, which, over time, are the major culprits of many chronic health conditions such as diabetes, high blood pressure and congestive heart failure (CHF).

Additionally, when individuals live in areas with increased crime rates, it can be more difficult to get appropriate exercise. If a neighborhood is unsafe, it becomes exponentially harder to incorporate exercise into a daily routine. There also may not be time to get sufficient exercise if working multiple jobs is required simply to make ends meet. In many cases, the same habits tend to be passed down from generation to generation. As children, we most often adopt the habits that were passed down to us from the adults in our lives. In this way, it can be difficult to break free from unhealthy cycles or to realize there is something to break free of.

For all of these reasons, diabetes takes on the role of something that cannot be conquered or defeated. Fortunately, with specific lifestyle changes, diabetes risk factors can be reduced and in those who already have it, adverse outcomes could possibly be mitigated.

Thoughts to Ponder:

- What two improvements could you start/change in regards to when it comes to meal planning?

- What does the current makeup of your plate look like? What is the percentage of carbohydrates, fats and proteins?

- What food group could you increase that would make your meals healthier?

CHAPTER 3:

The Current Barriers to Successful Care

Whether you're suffering with diabetes or are unknowingly living with prediabetes, there are three basic barriers in the way of successful management.

Awareness

The first hurdle that individuals face is a lack of awareness. Most people simply don't know that the foods they choose to put into their body and the lack of regular, physical activity are critical determinants of health. It's not that this information isn't out there and available to us. It has more to do with the fact that the message is not being explained in a way that meets everyone's health literacy levels.

We all know that we should eat healthy. It's common enough advice that we've all heard it before. The trouble is we don't know what "eating healthy" really means. Additionally, we feel relatively the same no matter what we eat. In fact, we feel better in some ways. We're not starving and experiencing hunger pains any longer, so the quick math is to simply eat what's filling. It's not like we eat a fast food burger or a slice of cake and feel any immediate impact on our health. We eat, the food tastes good, we have energy, what more could we ask for?

We don't grow up equating the food choices we make every day with actual health. The important part seems to be fulfilling the hunger in our stomachs, making sure everyone is fed with a paycheck that never seems to be enough, and then getting on with what's important. What we fail to stop and realize is that health is one of the most important things we can give ourselves.

Even as we come home from the doctor's office with a new diagnosis of diabetes, we still don't really understand what that means and how inextricably linked that is to our diet. Every food choice in our life has caused the current insulin control problem that we're now experiencing. Essentially, we overwhelmed our body and its ability to process food effectively. Now we have a broken system, and we have to treat it with extra care so that it doesn't hurt us.

One of the best things we can do as we learn to live with diabetes is to raise awareness about the disease. Share with family and friends that food choices do matter. They don't just matter theoretically or indirectly. They play a very important role in the blood sugar levels we maintain and are one of the direct correlations over time in regards to a diabetes diagnosis. The unhealthy, processed foods that you are stocking your cabinet with are no different than a pack of cigarettes was in relation to lung cancer twenty years ago. Although these are two completely different diagnoses that affect different organs, the common factor is that self-inflicted bad habits can lead to unplanned and unwanted diagnoses. When we make ourselves aware of this reality, we give ourselves the opportunity to do something about it.

Access

The second barrier to successful management is access. When you don't have access to healthy food or opportunities for exercise, it becomes much more difficult to integrate these things into your life. When you only have a certain denomination available with which to buy groceries, you don't spend that money on foods that don't go very far. You buy the cheapest items that can turn into filling meals. That might mean buying a large box of pasta and a jar of canned sauce. It might mean buying the cheapest and fattiest cuts of meat. It might mean skipping the fresh produce and going with easy-to-prepare items loaded with sodium and sugars.

If you shop in a grocery store that is stocked with every ingredient imaginable, even when your list includes obscure items, it can be difficult to imagine that food deserts exist. Unfortunately, these deserts are real. There are places where people literally don't have healthy choices, and they are forced to select whatever keeps them alive another day. Alternatively, sometimes grocery stores are many miles away from certain communities, and there are no public transportation options. This also results in a food desert.

The same is true when it comes to getting the proper exercise. Not everyone lives in a neighborhood that is safe to walk around in. Rather than risking their safety, individuals instead opt to stay inside. This might keep them alive, but it's not doing anything for their cardiovascular health. These realities have a real effect on overall wellbeing, including emotional and mental health in addition to the physical. Without access, prioritizing wellness is not just something that people can't get to on their exhaustive to-do lists, it's an unimaginable reality.

Acceptance

Acceptance is the final barrier to successful management. It's impossible to manage diabetes or prediabetes without accepting the reality of the disease. It can be very easy to deny, especially when there is no visible evidence that anything is wrong. Sure, your doctor might tell you that you have high blood sugar or an elevated A1C, but those assertions are almost meaningless to the point of being fictional. What does it matter if there is a lot of sugar in your blood if you are trying to come up with the money for the next mortgage payment? Why prioritize eliminating alcohol and sweets from your diet if you are worried about losing your job? Why worry about the impact of the free donuts available at work if you are simply happy to have breakfast?

The truth is that diabetes is a serious problem. It has huge repercussions for our quality of life, and taking it seriously is not a sign of weakness or a case of having skewed priorities. When our health is compromised, nothing else matters. If you're bed-ridden or losing limbs due to the progression of diabetes, your old priorities will very quickly mean very little. That's why it's so important to accept that there is a problem, that diabetes is a pernicious disease worthy of your undivided attention. When you prioritize your care and your health, you can significantly improve your life and the lives of those around you.

It doesn't help to get angry at the disease and write it off or pay it no mind. I've known many people who after their diagnosis decide they will simply try to get the better of diabetes. They'll cheat and say, "I can have a drink today," or "one dessert won't hurt." They might even respond with, "I'll just take a bigger dose of insulin." These people nearly always cause more damage. I know it isn't easy to completely revise your diet, seemingly away from all the good stuff that you grew up enjoying, but you can find joy in food again. It just might look a little different than what you're used to. Plus, I promise that once you start making some dietary changes, you'll start feeling healthier and more energetic so that those small dietary sacrifices will be worth it.

Despite these barriers, it is very possible to beat the sugar B.E.A.S.T. In the coming chapters, I'm going to provide you with some simple tips to effectively manage your diabetes and live a satisfying and complete life. No matter what your circumstances are, everyone has the ability to live well. It just might take a little more effort if you're facing any of the barriers we discussed earlier. The good news is that there is plenty of hope and with sacrifice, self-care and self love, a healthy life is completely within your reach.

Thoughts to Ponder:

- Have you ever been faced with the difficult decision of purchasing groceries or paying for medications? If so, how did you resolve this situation?

- Do you have a family member with the diagnosis of diabetes, who denies or does not believe they have it or that it is a serious condition? If so, what strategies related to behavior change may be incorporated to help move them forward in their diabetes management?

CHAPTER 4:

B – Behavior Changes

"Our behaviors reflect what we believe. If we want to change our behavior, we have to change our beliefs." ~ Patty Houser

If we never truly buy into the importance of diet, exercise and lifestyle on our health, it will be very difficult to make the necessary behavior changes to improve our quality of life. If we desire a different result, we have to start by changing our current behaviors and habits.

If we see dietary changes as futile, we won't make it a priority to eat differently. If we decide that exercise can't be that important, then we certainly won't carve out time to engage in it every day. If we don't believe that we play a vital role in our own wellness, then we won't take the initiative to self-advocate. Therefore, the first step is to shift what we believe. We have to see our actions in a different light than what we might be accustomed to. If we never saw our habits as consequential to our health, now is the time.

Intuitively, we all already know this. Imagine back to being a kid. If the walk home from school involved climbing up a large hill, and every day we got blisters from the long walk, we'd pretty quickly realize that we needed to change our behavior in some way. We might try to find another route that avoided the steep hill. We might try wearing different shoes that provided better traction for the walk home, or maybe we'd save up our chore money to buy a bike. We certainly wouldn't continue doing the exact same thing that only worsened our blisters and made the walk more difficult with each passing day.

Dealing with diabetes is similar. The primary difference is simply that we might not experience physical pain immediately after completing some of the less desirable behaviors, meaning the association between the behavior and the result would be less obvious. For that reason, we might not come to the conclusion of change as quickly, but eventually we would get there. Your doctors are likely telling you to make some changes. If you haven't been diagnosed with anything, your family history might indicate a need for change. Alternatively, you can probably tell based on your risk factors if behavior changes would be beneficial for you.

Behavior changes sound a lot worse than they are. After all, the only reason that you have a set of current behaviors is because somewhere along the line, you decided to engage in them. Over time, these behaviors became habits. Maybe you modeled the behaviors of your parents, maybe you adopted lifestyles similar to your friends and close contacts, or maybe you just sort of ended up with these behaviors by default. Adopting a new set of behaviors doesn't have to be dramatic. It's simply a conscious choice to do something new, something that is beneficial for your health, and something that is manageable to start and maintain.

At the beginning of the chapter, we eluded to changing your belief in order to change your behavior. That not only refers to a belief that your actions have impact, it also extends to having a belief in your diagnosis. Many people who are diagnosed with diabetes dismiss the diagnosis. They sort of shrug it off as unimportant or write it off as just another issue the doctor has decided to focus on. It is similar to being told we are overweight. We hear the words, and we might agree that we'd benefit by shedding a few pounds, but it certainly doesn't seem dire. If we are content with going up a pants size, then that's our own business. In some ways, a diabetes diagnosis lands in a similar fashion. Sure, we should ease up on the sugar; we've always known that, but is it really such a big deal?

Unfortunately, the answer is a resounding, YES!!! A diabetes diagnosis is very significant and is not something we should take lightly or write off. We have to truly believe that the condition is significant if we hope to make any lasting behavior changes. Diabetes should be seen as a very loud wake-up call. If you're told that your sugar levels put you in the prediabetes range that also needs to be taken very seriously. At the prediabetes level, you can still avoid a Type 2 Diagnosis, but that can't happen without some serious behavior changes.

Granted, if you are diagnosed with diabetes and you are overwhelmed or confused by the changes being asked of you, take a breath. It's okay to feel lost, especially initially. After all, an entire lifetime of habits has led you to this point, so you aren't expected to simply have all the answers the next day. However, if you are ready and open to learning, you'll do just fine. A big part of coping with a diabetes diagnosis is determined by your ability to adapt and a readiness to learn. If you already had all the answers, you might not be in this position, so no one is asking you to overhaul your entire life in a matter of a few short days.

It could be more helpful to think more long-term. You're not starting a new diet that you'll only have to adhere to for a month or two. You are being tasked with permanent lifestyle changes that both make sense in your daily life and that put your health first. Many African Americans struggle with a diabetes diagnosis because it doesn't fit into their current lifestyle, especially if they live in food deserts or have limited access to healthy food. Suddenly, it's not just their life that is more difficult, it's the lives of everyone around them. Affording better quality food and new, often expensive medications has repercussions on the entire family. By adding in new exercise routines or tacking on hours to what were formerly short grocery store trips can change the dynamic at home in ways that are difficult for other family members to adjust to. They may not understand why all of the changes are necessary.

So yes, behavior changes have repercussions. The positive is that once everyone involved overcomes the initial resistance, the benefits should far exceed the negatives. And in some ways, when one person in a family is diagnosed with diabetes, it's a great learning opportunity for everyone else. Even if others don't share the diagnosis, they might have other problems that are the result of the same bad habits. For example, a spouse might not have diabetes but might have high blood pressure or heart problems. In this way, adopting changes that help diabetes will have benefits for both partners.

The first step to knowing what changes to make, is to first understand what behaviors are problematic. We will get into many of these behaviors in the following chapters. Once the problem behaviors are determined, it's time to decide what to replace them with. The best way to do this is come up with SMART goals. SMART goals are Specific, Measurable, Attainable, Realistic and Time-Bound. The reason for this is best illustrated with a goal that isn't any of these things. For example, if you try to change your behaviors by deciding to "Be Healthier," you're not likely to make it very far. For starters, it's not specific. What does it mean to be healthier? It's also not measurable, so you have no way of knowing if you've achieved it. It might be realistic, but it's so vague we can't say for certain. And lastly, there is no time component. If something comes up, you can push that goal to the side for the night and indulge in some unhealthy behaviors.

A better goal might be something like, "Walk for 30 minutes every day for the next month." This goal is specific. You know exactly what needs to be done. It's measurable. If you have a phone and/or watch, you'll be able to check that you're walking for the allotted time each day. It's attainable and realistic in that it's not an impossible feat. You're not committing to something that you can't reasonably achieve. And lastly, there's a clear time component. Each day you need 30 minutes and you need to do that for one month. That's all very easy to track.

Once you have some goals like this set up for yourself, it's very easy to watch yourself make progress. People love to feel like they are making progress toward a goal. By mid-month, you'll be bragging to family members that you've been walking every day for two weeks. You'll be counting down the days and feeling accomplished and empowered. By the end, you'll likely be ready to set a new, possibly more ambitious goal. But if your goal had been vague, it would be long forgotten. You would have made no progress toward living better with your diabetes, and you'd likely be trapped in the same old habits.

Now that you understand a little about the importance of behavior changes and how to start going about them, let's dive into the most important change for someone diagnosed with diabetes: eating.

Thoughts to Ponder:

- What SMART goal can you set for your health and commit to today?

- Make a list of some potential behavior changes that you can make over the next 30 days.

- Do you have any hesitations when it comes to those changes? Explore those hesitations in more depth.

CHAPTER 5:

E- Eating Healthy

"I can't control everything in my life,
but I can control what I put in my body."

Eating healthy is of supreme importance in diabetes management. It's a practice that is beneficial for everyone, but for people living with diabetes it helps contribute to the additional benefits of blood sugar management, which in most cases will help manage hypo/ hyperglycemic symptoms, and also help to reduce the possibility of complications and damage. Secondly, it will help you get to a healthier weight. Not all people living with diabetes are overweight, but carrying extra weight creates additional problems. When your weight is reduced, you are also more likely to get better A1C results.

An A1C test measures the percentage of hemoglobin that is coated with sugar. This measure is a good indication of what your blood sugar levels have been over the past three months. Losing just 5 to 10% of your overall body weight could help you to reduce your A1C levels by 0.5%.

So, what is healthy eating really, and how can you ensure you're actually doing it? There are so many conflicting messages floating around on the Internet that it can be difficult to determine what you should be eating and what you shouldn't be eating. Add to that the various obstructions involved with obtaining and affording healthy food, and you'll feel defeated before you even begin.

In terms of eating healthy, there are some general guidelines I typically suggest to people. By keeping it simple in this way, it ensures that following this type of meal plan is manageable. Nothing is worse than to look at these eating changes as if you are going on a permanent diet. A diet is all about lack. It means we have to suddenly and drastically cut out all foods that are bad for us. In my opinion, that's a pretty heavy order. The plan that I recommend for people with diabetes, and which actually works wonders for anyone, including those with whom you share a household, focuses on eating more whole foods, less processed foods and saving your guilty pleasures for special occasions.

Eat More Real Food

Fresh food is always going to be more nutritious than boxed, canned, frozen and prepared food. The trouble is often fresh, whole foods are not available in certain neighborhoods and stores. If you're on a tight budget, you might be forced to purchase a lot of your food from dollar stores or other discount markets. These types of stores do not sell fresh items, and it can be tempting to substitute frozen meals for fresh. The trick is to know what foods make sense to stock up on at these discount stores and what you should really splurge on if possible.

Buy your canned beans, rice, olive oils and paper products, like napkins, aluminum foil and plastic bags at dollar stores to save money. But when it comes to ingredients that matter, buy real fruits and vegetables. Meat can be expensive, but you don't need to include meat at every meal. Incorporate protein from vegetarian sources and spread the meat options out throughout the week, especially if it strains your budget. Make vegetables and low starch carbs the centerpiece of your plate. Make meals more filling by adding nuts, seeds and healthy fats to your meal plan if this is not contraindicated for any of your other medical diagnosis/es.

What you may not realize is that real food is more filling than processed food. One chocolate chip cookie easily turns into an entire sleeve of cookies because there is not any nutritional value in those cookies, so your body is not satisfied. Mentally, you're happy because you're eating something sweet, but it's not providing lasting nourishment. The refined carbs cause your blood sugar to spike suddenly and quickly drop. As soon as it drops, you'll be hungry again. Eating real food provides you with fiber and other nutrients that slow down your digestion without raising your blood sugar. Meals loaded with protein, healthy fat and fiber will help you stay full longer.

You might also be thinking that as a person with diabetes you can't eat fruit. This is not true. It's important to focus on fruits with a low glycemic index, but you can and should eat fruit based on your nutritional needs. Apples, pears and berries are all great fruit choices in moderation. Be cognizant about where in the grocery store you are getting your fruit. The produce section is the best place to shop. For example, eating pears from a jar is not a great option because canned and jarred fruit often contains added sugars, which will only raise your sugar levels.

Ultimately, the closer a food is to how it appears in nature, the better it is for you to consume. If it's unrecognizable, covered in sauce and soaked in sugar, look for a better alternative. Once you can get into the habit of eating more real foods, you'll find it's not as difficult or time-consuming as you may have thought. Vegetables can be sautéed in olive oil and ready in just a few minutes. Rice can be cooked in a rice cooker with little attention. Eggs can serve as a protein when you don't have any meat in the house.

There are so many resources available online. If you are looking for affordable recipe ideas, the Internet abounds with meals that are healthy, delicious and affordable. Hopefully, by being creative and thinking outside of the box, you can come up with recipes that easily fit into your life; this will make it so that you are less reliant on processed foods. Plus, real foods taste better. By stocking up on healthier food choices, you'll also have less of the bad foods available in your cabinet and on your counter. When those foods aren't there, you won't be tempted to reach for them, and soon you won't even really miss them.

If you can get away with it, stop buying the processed items that you're eliminating from your diet for your family members as well. Get everyone on board with healthy eating. One perspective of your family members might be that they can still eat anything so they should be able to indulge in snacks and processed foods that they are accustomed to. Unfortunately, that's not really the way to look at it. These foods are not good for anyone. They cause a wide range of problems. The best meal plan for a person with diabetes is actually one that best serves everyone, and this shift in nutrition is a great opportunity for the entire family to up their health game. Remember, this is a lifestyle change, and this is the lifestyle that leads to lasting health. It's not about how long you can get away with eating candy bars and fast food. Eat real food, not food made in a building, and improve your quality of life.

Portion Control

Portion control is another great way to easily shift into a more diabetes-friendly eating pattern. When you eat too much, especially too many carbohydrates, it can cause your blood sugar to spike. Also, if it's beyond the amount of food you need, that energy can't be used and will be stored as extra weight. That's why it's important to be mindful of portion sizes.

One easy way to make sure that your portions are in line with what your body needs is to load your plate up with mostly vegetables rather than carbohydrates like pasta, rice or potatoes. Protein and healthy fats are both more filling than carbohydrates so when you eat more of those things, you will be fuller faster. When the bulk of your meal consists primarily of carbs, you won't feel full quickly and will end up eating more, raising your sugar. When possible and available, it is important to connect with a dietitian who can guide you on things like, calorie count, carbohydrate control and the necessary guidelines that are required to manage and maintain your health/meal planning needs.

Keep in mind that out in the world, portion sizes have grown uncontrollably. The bagel that you buy at the local shop has grown over the years so that it's no longer one serving size anymore. Restaurants serve you a plate of food that is not truly meant to be eaten at one sitting. One thing to consider may be to request a to-go box prior to eating your meal; set half aside in the container to take home with you and eat the other half. This way you can reduce your portion size and avoid eating the entire meal in one sitting. Even packaged foods available at the store often contain so many calories that they are divided into multiple servings if you look at the nutritional information on the back. For this reason, as Americans, we no longer naturally understand what an appropriate serving actually is. Try using smaller plates at home to avoid the temptation of filling up an extra large plate. Eat less protein and carbs and fill up that plate with non-starchy vegetables.

Plan Ahead

The smartest thing you can do as you're trying to adapt to a new way of eating is to sit down and plan your meals ahead of time. At the beginning of the week, decide what your meals will look like all week long, and then go to the store with a list of ingredients rather than just shopping spontaneously. Not only is this technique great for meal planning, it's also beneficial for your wallet. When you plan ahead, you have the opportunity to repurpose ingredients for different meals. This will help you use your fresh ingredients before they go bad so you're not wasting money on items you can't use.

If it makes sense to buy certain ingredients in bulk, you'll want to have a plan for using all of the ingredients. Learn to run your kitchen like a chef. When you have something that is about to go bad, utilize it in a meal. The more you do this, the better you'll get at it.

Planning ahead will prevent you from getting into dangerous food situations. These are times when you have nothing available. You let yourself get to the point where you're extremely hungry, and before you know it, you're indulging in something that isn't good for you because it was the easiest and fastest thing you could get your hands on. This is a practice that is best avoided. Always have healthier snacks on hand and easy options that you can whip up in an emergency. When you're prepared, it will be a lot more difficult to make poor choices.

Get Resourceful

If you live in a food desert or have little access to healthy options, I encourage you to get creative. Whatever your circumstances are, there are always options. There are food services that you can access online. These places will deliver food right to your door. If local options are not possible, you might want to start exploring online to see what other options are available to you. Your nutrition is too important. Don't resign yourself to what is around you. Figure out what you can do to improve your situation. If it means traveling a good distance to find a store with the ingredients you need, do it. Maybe that means that you have to buy more ingredients and then freeze items. Or maybe it means being resourceful with your budget so that you can afford transportation. Are there other things that you can give up in order to prioritize your nutrition? Can you cancel a television subscription or something else in order to put more money toward your health? Instead of spending lots of time watching television or playing video games, fill that time with activity or exercise.

On that note, let's move onto the next letter in our plan for managing diabetes. It's time to talk about activity and weight management.

Thoughts to Ponder:

- What's one food item which you eat regularly that you can replace with a healthier option?

- Do you meal plan? If not, write out what a sample week would look like for breakfast, lunch, dinner and snacks?

- Try grocery shopping with a list of specific ingredients? Does it feel different, take less time, feel satisfying?

CHAPTER 6:

A – Activity and Weight Management

"The only bad workout is the one you didn't do."

Activity is a critical component in managing diabetes successfully. The simplest explanation is that your body uses glucose for fuel, so when you engage in activity, especially after a meal, your body has the opportunity to use that fuel. This naturally lowers your blood sugar. One small study determined that walking just 10 minutes after a meal can lower your blood sugar by 22%. And the American Diabetes Association agrees that this effect can last for up to 24 hours or more after the actual exercise because muscle cells are using your insulin more efficiently and are continuing to utilize glucose even while at rest.

Put simply, when blood glucose is high, there are only two ways to reduce the sugar. Your body can either rely on insulin to use or store the glucose or your muscles can use some of this glucose while engaging in activity. Even just minimal exercise has positive effects, and when you are engaging in activity regularly, the effects are cumulative.

In addition, exercise helps reduce weight and the size of your fat cells. This is important because your insulin sensitivity improves when your fat cells are reduced in size. One study in the International Journal of Obesity showed that women who engaged in both diet and exercise reduced the size of abdominal fat cells by 18% compared to those who only focused on diet.[1] As always, consult your physician or medical professional before beginning an exercise routine or regimen.

---

[1] You, Tongjian, Murphy, K.M. Lyles, Mary, F. Demons, J.L. "Addition of aerobic exercise to dietary weight loss preferentially reduces abdominal adipocyte size." September 2006. International Journal of Obesity. 30(8):1211-6 DOI:10.1038/sj.ijo.0803245.

Physical Barriers

However, regardless of how important activity is in successful diabetes management, it remains a challenge for a large portion of the population. For those who don't live a safe neighborhood, regular and consistent exercise can be a problem. Instead of venturing out, it can be easier to stay inside or remain stagnant. This is an area for change. By avoiding exercise, it's contributing to an already epidemic problem. Mindset and education related to activity and weight management are two key areas that can inspire individuals to start moving more.

Before we can do anything, we have to understand the importance of exercise. If we can all get on board with the true value of activity, we can then start to find ways to prioritize it even if our situation is not conducive to outdoor exercise. If it is unsafe to walk in your neighborhood, you must figure out another solution. Perhaps that means joining a gym. Memberships are growing ever more affordable. If you can fit a membership into your budget, this is a great option. If not, another option might be to find a used piece of equipment online and get it set up in your house, even if it's in a basement, garage or other area in your household. You can find a lot of reasonably priced items on various online websites. Home exercise equipment is always evolving, meaning those who have purchased expensive items are incentivized to upgrade. That could mean an excellent opportunity if you don't mind using earlier models.

In addition, if your home environment is not the best for walking, then try visiting other local areas. Maybe the neighborhood where you work is safer than where you live. Try walking on your lunch break. You can also find local tracks or parks where you can engage in activity. Solicit friends and family to join you. This serves a dual purpose. If you can get members of your community to buy into the importance of exercise, it will help change the entire energy of your

Pubmed.

circle into one that is more focused on health. And for some people, having an accountability partner will allow them to show up and be responsible for completing their exercise workout. Also, there may be videos, how-to books or other materials that can be borrowed from the library. These are excellent places to look for resources that can assist you on your exercise journey.

Mental Barriers

On that note, many of us have mental barriers to exercise and activity that prevent us from getting up and moving on a regular basis. The predominant mental barrier that I've witnessed is peer pressure. When those around us don't prioritize exercise, it can be difficult to get motivated. If everyone in your household spends the day on the couch tethered to a phone, a computer, television or video game, it can be very difficult to be the outlier. That means all of your motivation has to come from yourself, the temptation to skip activity is increased and bad habits are reinforced.

What can you do if you are the only one in your circle interested in making positive change? Unfortunately, you have to be the one to lead the way. Being surrounded by others who don't value activity is not an excuse to engage in the same sedentary behavior. There are some tricks that might help. Instead of continuing to spend the bulk of your time in the presence of those who don't share your desire to be active, look for online groups or peers who also want to exercise. Join group classes, venture out of your existing circle, and make plans to get out. Don't get mired in your current comfort zone.

Furthermore, don't get hung up on your ability. You're not attempting to become an Olympic athlete. Your only goal in this step is to move more. Try not to psyche yourself into believing that you are not qualified to exercise or you don't have the ability. The goal is simply to put yourself in motion, raise your heart rate, use some glucose and lose weight. We can all do something. Try various things until you find activities that you enjoy best. Maybe it's walking, maybe it's a group class at the gym or maybe it's doing workout videos alone in your house. Often you won't know what you like best until you give it a try, and you might surprise yourself. Be open to possibility.

Emotional Barriers

There is a possibility that you've already attempted to incorporate more activity into your life, and you received negative feedback from those around you. They might have commented on the futility of your goal or found other unfair ways to discourage you. Remember simply by taking action and engaging in some sort of activity, you are changing the course of your life and health. If others don't like it or want to put you down for this, you've got to be strong. Do what you can in order to surround yourself with supportive people. And try to become resilient to the negativity as best you can.

Chances are the more active you become, the better you'll feel all around. Exercising releases endorphins, the "feel-good" hormone so you might find that the more active you are, the better you are at shrugging off the naysayers. As you start to feel better in your body and are successfully living with diabetes, you'll soon find that you want to add other healthy behaviors to your routine. You'll start to see how your former way of life was contributing to lethargy, depression and pain. Everything is connected, and it's empowering to see the results of your healthy actions. Depression may also be a barrier to getting started. It is important to have your depression assessed and treated. Don't let it be an excuse for why you can't get active. Exercise may be one of the interventions that can help you effectively find more balance in terms of your emotional wellbeing.

Next up we'll talk about the primary focus of every person living with diabetes – sugar. How do we monitor it and what does the monitoring mean?

Thoughts to Ponder:

- What's one activity you enjoy doing or would be interested in learning more about that would count as activity and movement?

- Has depression or another mental health issue stopped you from starting an activity for weight management?

- What are you proactively doing to manage your mental health and move forward?

CHAPTER 7:

S – Sugar Watch

"What is so dangerous about sugar is that it doesn't just impact us based on what we consume of it today, it rewires our brains to ensure that we will consume more of it tomorrow." - Dr. Susan Pierce Thompson

If you've living with diabetes, you likely are beginning to understand the role of sugar in the condition. However, it's not as simple as reducing sugar intake in your diet. As a person living with diabetes, your body's mechanism of reducing blood sugar via insulin is impaired. Insulin resistance occurs when your fat, liver and muscle cells no longer respond correctly to insulin. Because of this, sugar collects in the blood and causes damage to blood vessels. Having elevated levels of glucose in the blood over time acts much like a poison. It overworks the insulin-producing pancreas and can eventually cause permanent damage to the organ. The excess sugar also takes a toll on other organs and vessels.

This is why it's important that people with diabetes monitor their sugar levels regularly. It's very important to collaborate with your medical provider to discuss individual needs and the ranges that would be best for your target goals. If you are using insulin and the dosage is incorrect, it could cause your blood sugar to drop too low or remain too high. Low blood sugar symptoms include excessive sweating, hunger, feeling faint or fatigued, mental confusion, headaches and anxiety to name a few. High blood sugar symptoms could vary from person to person and can include things like fatigue, blurry vision, increased urination and feeling very thirsty. The goal is to keep your blood sugar within your target range as much as possible. As always, follow your medical professional's recommendations for your individual blood sugar levels/parameters.

Glucose monitors are tools that are used to manage blood sugar levels and can help you avoid the discomfort of either hypoglycemia (low blood sugar) or hyperglycemia (high blood sugar). Because different foods and types of exercise will have different effects on blood glucose, these monitors are an effective tool in developing healthy habits and staying away from things that cause extremes in blood glucose. [2]

Barriers to Consistent Glucose Monitoring

Understanding the Purpose of Monitors

One problem that I've found in patients is that they falsely believe that once their insulin dosage is established, they no longer need or can glean any value from a glucose monitor. This is especially true when affording the monitor is already a hurdle. If patients don't see a continued, tangible value, it can be difficult to reconcile the expense or inconvenience, and they will slowly discontinue use.

Glucose monitors serve an ongoing purpose in your diabetes management beyond simple insulin regulation. They help you to see how different foods and exercise impact your blood sugar. This is important because it puts the power back into your hands. One frustration for many of my patients is that they feel at the mercy of their diagnosis. A body that once could process the food it was given is no longer capable and making so many dietary adaptations can feel disempowering. The good news is that your choices still do play a role in your health, and by learning what increases and decreases glucose, it can empower you to take charge of your health. When we understand what's going on with our body and how things like food and exercise affect it, we tend to make better decisions. In addition, not all food affects people the same. A food that causes your blood

---

[2] Karter AJ, Parker MM, Moffet HH, Ahmed AT, Ferrara A, Liu JY, Selby JV. Missed appointments and poor glycemic control: an opportunity to identify high-risk diabetic patients. Med Care. 2004 Feb;42(2):110-5. doi: 10.1097/01.mlr.0000109023.64650.73. PMID: 14734947.

sugar to spike might not have the same effect in someone else. In this way, you can't rely solely on general guidelines. You have to see for yourself what foods work best in your body.

When your doctor tells you that drinking alcohol or eating desserts is off limits or should be reduced, it can sound like an unfair restriction; but when you understand how consuming those things can cause fluctuations to your glucose to a point that is difficult for your body to process there is a stronger motivation to adhere to better habits.

Monitoring glucose could be an important tool for everyone. It would offer more understanding about what certain foods really do when they enter the body. Having diabetes is the result of a lifetime of eating without this understanding. You don't have to view your diagnosis as a punishment. Glucose monitoring provides a window into a mechanism that we, as a culture have spent years overlooking. We can view glucose tracking instead as a way to have more autonomy over your health. There is no good or bad. There is only information, which segues nicely into the next barrier.

Judgment

Many people stop monitoring glucose because they are discouraged when they see numbers that are out of range. The other side of the "more control" or "more autonomy" coin is that when testing regularly, people are exposed to more data and can easily take poor results to be their fault. Maybe they are not being diligent enough, or are eating the wrong foods and their body is not cooperating. The result is they end up feeling bad about themselves after every test, and so they stop checking.

It's important not to think of glucose monitoring like taking a test at school. It's not a measure of aptitude or effort on your part. Think of it more like filling up a tire. You check the pressure of your tires to make sure that it's not too high or too low, but you don't berate yourself if the psi is out of range. You simply react accordingly. You either add more air when it's low or you release some if you overfilled it. Blood sugar is a gauge of our glucose level at a particular moment in time – nothing more. It tells us what's happening on a cellular level and offers guidance as to what we should do next, but it's not a measure of any lasting quality. If the emotional component is a hurdle for you, try thinking of your glucose levels more like you think about your tire pressure. There doesn't have to be any judgment.

Cost

Cost is a big factor in both glucose monitoring and medication management. Glucose monitoring can be done via a continuous glucose monitor, which provides continuous access to blood sugar numbers or by using a blood glucose meter, which requires providing blood samples at key points during the day. In terms of medications, cost will determine the delivery style of your medication, which can be through oral medications, injections, or insulin delivery systems such as pumps. A significant portion of diabetes management comes down to what things cost, what is covered by insurance and whether those costs fit into a patient's life and budget. Generally, what I find is that if a cost can be avoided and it doesn't cause a visible or palpable difference in everyday life, patients won't adhere, the condition will go unchecked, and will likely progress until the symptoms are noticeable.

I typically recommend using whatever glucose monitors are covered by your insurance, but for many people insurance is not an option. Other times insurance covers only a portion of what is needed. When these hurdles arise, continued use quickly becomes a luxury that can't be maintained. Without coverage, patients need to purchase the glucose meter, lancets and testing strips themselves. Blood sugar needs to be checked multiple times throughout the day, which means replacements are needed regularly. These costs can quickly add up and often the answer is to simply reduce or avoid testing altogether. Many patients feel fine physically so erroneously decide that there is no point in continuing to test. The added stress of trying to take on that cost simply isn't worth it.

This is not a strategy I advise, but when the choice is between putting food on the table and buying more lancets and glucose strips, the choice is pretty obvious. However, I'd like to stress the importance of prioritizing your health once again. There are affordable testing options available to you even if you do not have insurance. You can also check with your employer to discuss what options are available for diabetes management or other chronic condition management. In some communities there may be local agencies that help with diabetes testing supplies for people managing their diabetes.

Many of my patients have little trouble rationalizing an unhealthy splurge purchase once a month. It's easy to justify a bottle of wine or some items from the bakery that would not be beneficial for your blood sugar, but it's often much harder to justify spending a similar amount of money on glucose testing strip refills. If you swap out an expense like this in your budget, it benefits you twofold. You are buying something needed for your health and you're avoiding something that would negatively affect your health. Over time, the benefits of managing your health and hopefully thwarting some of the dangerous effects of high blood sugars will be worth it.

In my experience, a large part of the problem with managing the cost comes from the mental barrier that we have in place. When we are spending money so that we can test for a single molecule in our body, it can seem futile, especially since the test is only a measure and not a cure or remedy. There are so many other pressing needs that it even seems self-indulgent or extraneous. Trust when I tell you that this is not true. Diabetes is a condition that is all about the details. Minimizing the amount of time that excess glucose is circulating in your blood is the difference between living a healthy life and suffering complications. The information gleaned from glucose monitoring is not trivial, so if there is a way to make it work in your budget, let's make it happen.

Stigma

Another barrier that I see people struggling with is the stigma attached to glucose monitoring. Testing your glucose levels is most helpful when done at multiple intervals throughout the day, often in relation to eating meals. This frequency easily begins to interfere with daily life. Many people are hesitant to do the testing in front of others and find it cumbersome to carry around the needed supplies. Because of all the equipment it takes to test regularly, my patients often report being self-conscious. They wonder what others will think of them or they worry they will make others uncomfortable.

Having diabetes in general comes with its own stigmas. Because it's seen as a lifestyle disease, meaning that it is caused by unhealthy habits, many people feel as though the condition itself is a judgment on their behavior. Testing in front of other people brings those emotions to the forefront. For this reason, people tend to skip tests if it interferes with their life in any way. Again, this is not an advisable position to take as it only further hurts your health. It's understandable to want to refrain from testing as it can deter others, but instead of avoiding it altogether, try to find some other less intrusive solution. You can be discreet without sacrificing your health.

There may be little you can do about your diagnosis and your past lifestyle, but you can definitely get yourself on a revised path now that you understand more about what's going on in your body. Instead of letting the existing stigma rule you, try taking a more proactive mentality. Be open and direct about your condition but be just as direct about what you're doing about it. If that includes using glucose monitors or insulin pumps, so be it. As a society, we are just now beginning to truly understand how much of a role the typical American diet has played in causing such a large proportion of the population to have diabetes. You don't have to bear the weight of that reality alone. There is more support for diabetes than ever before. Let's lean into that side of the stigma and focus on improving our health moving forward.

The Sweet Spot

I hope you're beginning to understand how important it is to prioritize your health and the resources that are available to support you on this journey. I understand completely all of the reasons that would deter you from acquiring the tools you need, but the cost of not making this effort is far worse. Diabetes is manageable. It's a disease that is all about making sure that your sugar levels stay in a healthy range. The only way to know if this is happening is by checking consistently. It may be inconvenient. It is definitely costly without insurance. And it can be frustrating that you have to shoulder the cost and energy to do something that your body should be able to handle on its own. Unfortunately, this is your reality. The good news is that you still have a lot of control, and with control, you can change your trajectory. Diabetes does not have to be something that defeats you. Think of it like a game if that helps. The only way to get the upper hand in this battle is to understand how your opponent plays. When you understand how your opponent is going to try to outsmart you, you can take steps to prevent this from happening. That's what you're doing in this Sugar Watch phase. You're beating diabetes at its own game. Use the tools at your disposal to keep your sugar levels in check. Whenever a hurdle arises that wants to get in the way of you and what you need to do to manage your diabetes, find a way around it. There is always a solution.

Thoughts to Ponder:

- What barriers have you faced in managing your blood sugar levels?
- Have you ever been concerned about people watching you monitor your blood sugar in public?
- What specific concerns do you have about monitoring?

CHAPTER 8:

T - Tackling Medication Management

"Let food be thy medicine and medicine be thy food." - Hippocrates

When you have diabetes, it's often not as simple as accepting your diagnosis, going home and adapting your diet and behavior. Treating and managing diabetes typically requires a plethora of medications in addition to any mindset obstacles. This might include oral medications, injectables, insulin and insulin pumps. Antihypertensives might be required to lower your blood pressure and diuretics might be prescribed to help with fluid retention. These medications might be required in addition to other medications treating related issues like weight loss, cholesterol or hypoglycemia.

For many patients, it is overwhelming to not only deal and manage the sheer plethora of medications, but to then afford all the associated costs. In some ways, diabetes is easily treated and managed, but only if there is a perfect storm of circumstances allowing for unrestricted medication, monitoring and insurance coverage. It's in large part due to the barriers we'll discuss below that patients end up neglecting or opting out of the required care, medication and appointment follow-ups they need to get a firm handle on the disease.

I'd liken the situation to the ease with which we see celebrities maintain their physical fitness levels. It's no wonder celebrities seem to effortlessly stay fit with the entourage of personal trainers, life coaches and personal chefs they have at their disposal. With all the needed resources and tools, even for a difficult task, are readily available and at your disposal, it's easy to adhere to strict regimens. But when getting even the most basic medication or monitor requires jumping through hoops, it's easy to see why many individuals end up failing when it comes to their care plan.

Diabetes management is similar to the above scenario in that it would all be very easy to manage if there weren't so many obstructions in the way for regular people to simply get the care they need. The more underserved the community, the more difficult this becomes. I can't single-handedly change that disparity, but I can shed some light on the problems. Hopefully, with a little bit of awareness, it can help you to advocate for yourself and make the small changes that could mean the difference between health and disease.

Let's dig a little deeper into the things that are preventing people from complying with the prescribed medications.

Insurance Coverage

Without insurance, the cost of insulin, in addition to any other medications required for care, quickly becomes very expensive. Even with insurance, the cost can still add up to unmanageable numbers. Many patients simply can't afford this cost, and so they naturally try to ration their insulin. They will attempt to get away with using less. This is dangerous from a health perspective as it can cause complications and even hospitalization, but many feel as if they have no choice.

With the cost of insurance prohibitively high, there doesn't seem to be many good solutions available. My suggestion is to scour the Internet for resources and discount programs that will help with the cost. You can also try to see if there are generic medications that are comparable to the ones you've been prescribed. Using generic medications will cut down on costs over time without sacrificing health.

Another option is to seek out government assistance, but this comes with its own barriers. Many times, individuals don't meet the income requirements for this option. To actually afford the exorbitant cost of these meds however, they'd have to make way over the income requirement. They are instead stuck in the gray area in between where support is not an option and cost is prohibitively high. Unfortunately, many people, including the working poor fall into this category.

Access to Care

The lack of insurance tends to lead to another big problem, and that's lack of care. Without coverage, individuals don't have many options when it comes to getting treated. They tend to wait until something significant happens and then end up in the emergency room. Diabetes is a condition that must be managed early and regularly. Waiting until you notice complications is not the best approach, but many individuals feel like there is no other option available to them. Even if they were to learn that they had diabetes, it would mean an onslaught of monthly expenses that are far too much for them to handle. To avoid this, they simply stay away from the doctor, which is easy to do without insurance, rather than to manage the costs of those visits.

If you can recognize that getting care is a top priority, you can start to explore alternative options. Maybe you need to change jobs to something that provides healthcare. Maybe there are resources online that you can tap into. You won't know until you start looking. One option is to look into community clinics. These establishments often have various payment plans or sliding scales to assist with payment. There are also Primary Care Offices that offer member subscription plans where you can purchase a plan and receive care based on your medical needs. Whatever you do, you can't bury your head in the sand and lean into the lack of access. Somehow, you have to figure out how you can get your needs met.

Follow-Up Appointments for Prescriptions

More often than not, if you're not going to the doctor regularly due to cost or access, it's unlikely that you will follow up for maintenance appointments. These are some of the most important moments in your care. It's one thing to receive a diagnosis, but after that, the game becomes management. The only way to manage your condition well is to do so in conjunction with your medical provider. The body is a fickle thing and there are a great deal of variables that play a role in your response to medication, meal planning and exercise. You need an expert to help you navigate all of this information. Diabetes management is a team effort, and there are multiple players on your team. These individuals may include an endocrinologist, a primary care provider (PCP), nurse practitioner (NP), registered nurse and/or a licensed practical nurse, certified diabetes care and education specialist (CDCES), a registered dietitian, social worker, and a pharmacist just to name your starting lineup. As your needs change and adjustments are made, you also may need an exercise physiologist, community health worker (CHW), podiatrist, ophthalmologist, cardiologist and other specialists to continue to manage your care.

Failing to attend follow-up visits is not only due to cost. Sometimes patients don't see the need and therefore have difficulty justifying the time off work needed, the money toward transportation, potential childcare etc. I've met patients with insurance that will cover the visit, perhaps with only a small co-pay, but they still skip the appointment because they decide it's unnecessary. Don't slip into this mindset. The more oversight and information you can have in your journey with diabetes, the better results you're going to have.

Transportation

This is one we often don't think about, especially if we're used to having our own transportation or being close to public transportation. For many individuals suffering with diabetes, transportation is a big problem. Some individuals start out strong by relying on family members, but eventually they start to feel like too big of a burden. They slowly begin to fall out of adherence and eventually cease appointments altogether.

Others never had any source of reliable transportation. They may not live near public transportation and can't afford other means. These individuals quickly opt out of care because they can't make it happen. If transportation is a problem for you, it's so important to find a solution. See if there is anyone you can barter with or look online for local options or groups. Maybe there are ways to conduct telemedicine appointments and get most of your medications/supplies delivered so that you are not relying on outside transportation all the time. Again, once you start making your health a priority, you'll have the motivation to get creative with any obstacles you encounter.

Difficulty Taking Pills/Medications

As we all know, taking regular medication is not easy. Amidst all of your current responsibilities, adding a list of pills or medications to the list can be a challenge. It's important to take your medications as recommended by your medical provider, but life does seem to get in the way. To successfully manage diabetes, it's important that medication management becomes a priority. If it means getting one of those pill containers with the days of the week labeled on it or setting alarms and alerts on your phone, it's something that has to be done.

Blood sugar is a constantly changing metric. When it's high, there is potential for it to cause damage to various areas in your body. The primary medications used in diabetes work to keep this blood glucose in balance, and that is done best when taken at the appropriate times. Other medications that you're taking might be less time-sensitive, but regardless, you need to make taking them a habit.

When your schedule is hectic or constantly changing, it can be easy to miss a dose. It's up to you to set up a system that works within your life. It might seem like an inconvenience or you might resent that you're restricted in this way, but trust me, it will be a bigger inconvenience if your diabetes progresses.

Medication Risks/Benefits

Some patients display hesitancy toward the medications because of unwanted side effects or risks, and because they are unsure of the benefits. It's one thing to be hesitant or curious about what is being prescribed. Ask as many questions of your medical provider as you can think of. It's never a good idea to blindly take a medication that you are unsure about. However, if you find that you skip or miss doses because of your concerns, reach out. There might be other alternatives that are a better fit for you. You also might find that you had been misinformed about the dangers whether it be through others' experiences or what you've read online. Don't hesitate to voice your concerns. Be honest about what you're experiencing, but make sure to get all the facts so that you can make the best decision for you.

Familial/Friend Adverse Reaction

It's important to remember that diabetes is a very personal disease. Not everyone with diabetes is going to have the same experience. It's very possible that a food that causes your blood sugar to skyrocket has no effect on the next person. That's why glucose monitoring is so important. It helps you to see how you react to different stimuli. Some medications will work well for you, but won't work well for a family member or friend. There are many factors that determine this. Again, it's fine to have concerns, but the best thing to do is to bring them up with your medical provider. That person has insight into your history and system and will have the best feedback as far as what protocol you should follow.

Cost Adherence

For some patients, there is a time right after their diagnosis where they are scared. They learn about the condition, and they are motivated to do whatever is recommended regardless of the cost. Taking on high costs for a few months might be manageable. It's also at this stage that a person might utilize any credit they have available. But eventually, the costs start to add up at an intolerable rate. The fear starts to wear off, and the burden of the cost becomes too much. In these instances, people simply stop adhering to their doctor's advice.

It can be difficult to take medications that are for maintenance purposes only. Our minds like to see results, so when we are prescribed an antibiotic for strep throat and the sore throat goes away in a few days, we feel like we got something for our money. We bought a solution. With diabetes, the medications are helping the body to carry out processes that it used to be able to do on its own. We keep taking the medications, but we don't get better. It's just more of the same. And it's not just a few bucks here and there. It adds up fast. This may be one reason so many people don't stick with it. The best defense for this barrier is to understand the true cost of stopping medications. Things only get worse when you try to go off your medications.

The bottom line is that managing medications is of supreme importance in handling diabetes, but as you can see there are a great deal of obstacles in the way. If it was as simple as getting some aspirin at the drugstore, diabetes might not be such an overwhelming diagnosis. The truth unfortunately is that managing diabetes well comes with a lot of costs, effort and understanding. It's a full lifestyle change, and requires an overhaul of your financial, dietary and physical habits in order to best serve you.

Thoughts to Ponder:

- What has been the biggest obstacle in managing your diabetes diagnosis?

- What have you done to overcome these obstacles? How did you arrive at your solution?

CHAPTER 9:

Case Study

In order to illustrate more clearly how the B.EA.S.T. methodology can help a person living with diabetes, let's take a look at a case study. You may find some similarities in your own situation, and from this may be able to picture the sorts of changes that could be important for you to make in your own life.

Thelma is a 52-year old African American female who is married with two children. She has a 14-year old son and a 22-year old daughter. Thelma was diagnosed with gestational diabetes during her pregnancy with her son and then six years ago was diagnosed with Type 2 diabetes. Since high school, she's been struggling with her weight, but over the last ten years, she has gradually put on an extra fifty pounds. She works in an office setting, and most of her day is spent sitting at a computer. She walks occasionally on her lunch break for about ten minutes, but her breathing has become more strained and she is often short of breath after these walks. Her commute is an hour and a half round-trip, and she takes the train both ways.

Her husband, Bernard works the night shift and rarely gets a chance to eat meals with the family, often relying on quick meals he picks up on the way to work; he had a stroke five years ago. Together they are in the process of purchasing another vehicle since their previous car broke down and is beyond repair. They are both working hard to make ends meet. Covering the cost of Thelma's meds is a considerable strain on the finances as they try to afford food, rent and other necessities. As a family, they are considered part of the "working poor," and do not qualify for governmental assistance for food or supplemental medical coverage based on their income. Unfortunately, they make $50.00 over the income limit. The "working poor" are people who spend 27 weeks or more in a year in the labor force either working or looking for work, but whose incomes fall below the poverty level. Poverty thresholds are the income dollar amounts used by the U.S. Census Bureau solely as a statistical yardstick to determine a household's poverty status. They are issued each year in September and are the basis for determining the national poverty rate. [3]

Thelma and Bernard are both dealing with health issues that require medications; sometimes this means they must skip their medicine to make sure bills are paid and groceries are purchased for the family.

Thelma and Bernard decided to work the B.E.A.S.T. Methodology. In doing so, they started with Behavior Changes. In the spirit of change, they decided to focus on accepting their medical diagnoses. Although neither of the children had been diagnosed with diabetes or any other chronic medical conditions, they were both overweight. Thelma and Bernard decided to take the family in another direction. They decided they would all try to lose weight with the assistance of a local community counselor/therapist. This counselor advised them to set SMART (Specific, Measurable, Attainable, Realistic and Time Bound) Goals. The family realized that when they all worked together, they were more effective at hitting milestones.

Initially, when Thelma was diagnosed with her diabetes, she became depressed. This caused her to stop walking at work and resulted in her gaining an additional five pounds. After adopting the new family Behavior Changes, she realized that this was not the answer. It was time to focus on Eating Healthy as part of the methodology. She resumed her walking and started researching healthier meal choices. Although her family lived in a food desert and the nearest grocery store was about 30 minutes away, she decided to look into alternatives. What she came up with turned out to be a pleasant surprise. Several of the local churches sponsored food pantries in her area, and one of the churches started a

---

[3] "Who are the Working Poor." Data from the Bureau of Labor Statistics. Center for Poverty and Equality Research. University of California Davis.
https://poverty.ucdavis.edu/faq/who-are-working-poor-america

Farmer's Market where she could receive a voucher to pick up fruits and vegetables twice a month. The amount of food she was eligible to receive was based on her household size. Ultimately, even though her community lacked access to the grocery store and many of the residents and neighbors did not have transportation, the farmer's market and food pantry provided her access to the groceries she needed for her family.

Thelma and Bernard started to work on the Activity and Weight Management component next. Over time, some of the churches recognized the need and desire within the congregation to offer fitness classes. With growing interest levels and waivers being signed, Thelma and fellow church members were able to participate in evening and weekend classes. Her children were also able to participate in the classes. Over time, the exercise helped improve Thelma's mental wellbeing, increased her physical stamina, and provided a fun outlet for her family.

In addressing Sugar Levels, Thelma realized that she became disinterested in monitoring her glucose levels early in her diagnosis. After noticing increased urination and developing boils under her arms and in her genital areas, she had a wakeup call. She realized she needed to pay more attention to her blood sugar numbers and committed to checking them daily. Initially, she could not afford the testing supplies, but after discussing her concerns with her doctor and nurse practitioner, she was able to switch to a more affordable glucose monitor. Shortly after, she started noticing trends in the morning before eating and also two hours after the start of a meal. She was able to witness the effect exercise had on her blood sugar levels and learned that by eating a snack prior to exercising, she could prevent post exercise blood sugar lows.

For years, Thelma and Bernard had the regrettable task of figuring out which bills would get paid, which medications would be purchased and what they had to make do without. As they addressed the Tackling

Medication Management pillar into their regimen, they reflected on an unfortunate incident. In Bernard's situation, taking medication literally meant life or death. He was on a blood thinner since his stroke diagnosis and needed this medication to prevent another stroke or blood clot.

Bernard stopped taking his blood thinner after a couple months because he had an uncle that passed away and happened to be on the same medication. Bernard believed there was a correlation between his uncle's death and the medication; his response was to stop the medication. Unfortunately, after skipping his medication for a few months, he ended up having another stroke, which left him with right-sided weakness. Thelma and Bernard ended up scheduling an appointment with their PCP and discussed their concerns surrounding the medication usage, prescription costs and indications for use. The doctor connected them with a pharmacist at their local drug store, who provided them with prescriptions that would be covered at a lower price based on a three-month supply. With these new changes, Thelma and Bernard were able to free up money to purchase the new car that they so desperately needed. It also allowed them more room in their grocery budget.

This is an example of how a family who was struggling under the weight of their diagnoses were able to make their lives work just by being creative, resilient and making small but effective changes. But this methodology is not like a pill or quick fix. It's all about behavior, daily choices and committing to a change in lifestyle. In other words, it's a journey. But what happens when life gets in the way, and we fall off the wagon, so to speak. Well, that happened to our now-thriving family.

The COVID-19 Pandemic came in and shocked the world. Thelma's stress levels increased significantly when the Pandemic first arrived, and within a few months, she had family members and friends pass away. She became fearful and started to binge-eat. She soon lost track of her medications and missed several days of her dosages. Her blood sugar slowly became elevated and she started to gain weight. Essentially, she lost her way. Thelma and Bernard eventually had to stop, regroup and go through the process of making changes again. They had to remember what they had learned and implement some good habits regardless of what was happening in the world around them. They both made a conscious effort to get back on track and used their faith to do so. They reached out to their church family and prayed. They had open conversations about what they would do as a family to protect themselves throughout the pandemic, but they also realized that whatever they did, they would have to do it one day at a time. By thinking small and simple, they were able to find their way back onto a healthy path again.

CHAPTER 10:

Conclusion

As you hopefully have learned, diabetes is not a curse or a death sentence, but it is a serious condition that requires the proper attention. Living with diabetes successfully requires a mental shift that's different from what you might be used to. It's not a condition where the solution is cut and dry – *If you have it, take this pill and continue as normal.* Living well with diabetes requires a change in lifestyle.

Zooming out a bit, human beings are not living in a natural habitat that is ideal for us. We didn't evolve to eat the mainstream diets that we're currently indulging in. It's only been over the last 70 years or so that we've been consuming as many carbohydrates, processed foods and sugars as we are now. We are only just beginning to recognize what this is doing to our health. Diabetes is just one of a laundry list of diseases that are lifestyle related. Obesity, heart disease, stroke, high blood pressure and others are plaguing citizens, and those in underserved areas are taking the brunt of the blow.

Part of the reason for this is due to lack of access and resources. As our society learns more about what we should be eating and how we should be caring for ourselves, those in underserved areas are typically the last to know. The food available at their local markets doesn't change with the latest health information. In this way, we become mired in our situations. The things we have access to are the very things that are making us sick in a lot of cases.

The problems that brought us to our current situation are vast and deeply embedded. I do believe there is a hope that we can change things around, but my more pressing concern is helping individuals who are currently just trying to keep their heads above water. It all starts on the individual level. We have got to get serious about our health, and a diabetes diagnosis is a perfect place to start. Instead of looking at your diagnosis as something bad that's happening to you, there is room to look at it as an opportunity. It's almost like – enough is enough. It's time to open our eyes, take control of our health and start making smart decisions not just for ourselves, but for our children. It starts with understanding there is a problem, recognizing what's causing it and making changes that will take us down a new path.

A big reason why diabetes outcomes are so negative is due to all of the barriers I mentioned earlier. When we hear the diagnosis and then learn what it's going to take via money, willpower, and effort to keep it at bay, it almost feels like a losing battle. There's no way to win. This book is meant to show you the light. There is definitely a way forward that can be fulfilling, satisfying and doesn't mean that you're thinking about your condition 24/7. By changing the way, we think and being purposeful about the small choices we make on a daily basis, we can thrive. Diabetes does not have to wreck our health, our finances or our spirit. And when we live our lives in this way, we inspire the next generation to make smarter decisions for themselves. We are paving the way for a better future.

This book really only just touches on some of the changes that can empower you to successfully manage your diabetes. As I mentioned, diabetes is a personal condition, so every case is different. If you're looking to reform your life and are ready to manage your diabetes instead of letting your diabetes manage you, then I'm here for you. I work with individuals in all facets of the condition. Whether you're struggling with affording your medications or if the food restrictions have you depressed and resentful, I'm here to help. Please don't hesitate to get in touch and continue moving forward in your diabetes management.

To learn more about our educational offerings that will provide solutions in your Diabetes Journey, feel free to visit our website or send an email. We look forward to sharing in your growth and health victories along the way. Moving Forward with Diabetes Management, LLC

https://www.mfdmllc.com

info@mfdmllc.com

- National Diabetes Statistical Report 2020 Estimates of Diabetes and Its Burden in the United States. US Diabetes of Health and Human Services. Center for Disease Control and Prevention

- Prochaska and DiClemente's Transtheoretical Model of Change - Exploring your mind.com

- About Social Determinants of Health (SDOH) (cdc.gov)

- What is diabetes? | CDC

www.ingramcontent.com/pod-product-compliance
Lightning Source LLC
Chambersburg PA
CBHW060644280326
41933CB00012B/2142